Best practices in
Toddler
Discipline
from **1 to 5**
without tantrums

Effective Strategies for
Developing and Helping your Child

Mary Simmons

Here's your bonus

<<   http://marysimmonsbook.com/home/   >>

Table of Content

Preface

This book is dedicated to all responsible parents considering all the stress they go through and the work they put into ensuring the growth and development of their kids (physically, mentally, and spiritually) are achieved adequately.

Kids can sometimes behave bad (a lot of times); it is the job of parents to keep their kids' behaviors in check. Certain measures are required to curb the many bad habits exhibited by these kids in order to prevent these habits from becoming dominant parts in the body of the kid's personality and character.

A lot of work has been put into writing this book to help parents go through the hard task of parenting. I hope the aim of this book is achieved.

Introduction

Do you find it difficult knowing how to discipline your child? You don't want to be too harsh and at the same time, you don't want to be taken for granted by your kid when taking disciplinary measures on him/her, thereby making you one of the numerous parents who find themselves in this large group of "disciplinary actions clueless parents." Well, worry no more because you have finally got the solution in your hands, it is now up to you and only you if you want to enjoy your parenthood because after reading this book, you will learn how to handle, manage, and correct your kid's wrongdoings.

I'm not yet a parent. Even if you do not have kids yet, you are hoping to have one, or more, right? If yes, then we can all agree to the fact that nobody is perfect enough to say **"I don't need this book,"** well, you are free to say that, but only if you are prepared to live your whole parenthood as a nightmare, **why?** Because there is no such thing as a perfect child-who does not give you trouble at all, at one point or the other, your kid will surely give you some trouble, and you will need the right measures to tackle them adequately. Measures which might be hard to get instinctively. This is the reason this book looks to give you a free and easy access to the right methods by which you can discipline and correct your kid(s).

There is a whole lot of information waiting for you in this book, so I will advise you to pay attention and hold on to every little detail you can find. With this book, it is only a matter of time before you move from "being clueless" to "being enlightened," enlightened to know the different measures to be taken to correct every form of misconduct exhibited by your kid(s).

"Train up a child in the way he should go: when he is old, He shall never depart from it."

Part One
Parental Education

Meaning

What Is Discipline?

The essence and importance of discipline in a person's life can never be over-emphasized. Discipline entails both preventive and corrective measures which can be implemented aggressively or non-aggressively. Discipline can be self-oriented and between a higher and a lower figure, in the shape of parents-children, bosses-employees, and the likes.

Toddler discipline

Discipline can be exercised both aggressively and non-aggressively, but in the case of toddlers, the aggressive kind of discipline is never a good idea. Apart from the fact that it is unpleasant, it also never works. Toddler discipline is a set of measures taken to prevent the shortcomings in kids' behavior and character that kids might have in the future (when they are grown). What you plant into your kids, behaviorally, is what will grow with them as they grow up. Toddler discipline, in other words, can be the process by which you train your kids and show them the right manner at which they are expected to act in their day-to-day activities. Toddler discipline needs some careful measures taken, if you don't get professional advice, you may get it wrong, you need to know what you are doing when trying to discipline your kids and, in fact, throughout your parenthood.

Now let's see what this book has for us as we head into chapter one.

What is Your Parenting Mission?

Your mission as a parent over your kids consists so much that it makes it hard to pick out which is most important, but at the end of the day, you want to make sure that all the trainings and teachings you have given to them shapes them positively and helps them become better people. I am going to talk to us about some of them.

- **Making sure that your kids have and display moral values.** Moral values are a set of values that helps us differentiate between good and bad. They are generally a set of principles that we must follow to ensure peaceful living and maintain good relationships with the people around us. Examples of moral values include reliability, kindness, honesty and integrity, responsibility, respect for self and others, decency, et cetera. You have to make sure that you impart these values in your kids in order to build in them, acceptable personalities. Having moral values, in other words, can be described as being disciplined.

- **Help them become independent.** This is another goal you should want to achieve as a parent. Believe me, it is satisfying to watch your kids doing some things by themselves, but this cannot be achieved when you're always helping them do everything. You need to allow your kids to handle some things by themselves, this makes them self-dependent, boosts their confidence, and improves their problem-solving skills, another advantage is that it gives them high self-esteem. It is true that watching your kids spend twenty minutes doing what you would have done for them in two is exhausting, you still have to allow them to. Which might lead to time-wasting problems like if you let your kids brush their own teeth in the morning and it causes you to be late for work, what you do is to try and create more time by maybe waking them up earlier than usual, trust me, it gets better. Patience is key.

- **Sound health.** This, I can say, is conventional, you don't need an expert's advice to know that you have to ensure your kids are hale and hearty. Be sure to notice any slight uncommon symptoms in your kids and immediately take them to the medical center for a professional review. Don't be surprised that illness can cause behavioral changes in your kids, for example, they are usually cheerful and playful kids then suddenly changes and becomes abnormally dull, you should consult a pediatrician and be sure that they are okay. Also, make sure you read books on kids' health so that you will have a better idea on how to care for your kids' health. They can function only when they are healthy. Health is wealth.

- **Help them achieve.** As a parent, from the birth of your kids, you should start to take notice, what they like and dislike, the areas they are naturally good at, when you spot what your kids are good at, and you help them improve, you are already setting your kids on the right path. People like Ben Carson, Serena, and Venus Williams give great credit to their parents today for being pivotal in making them the success they have turned out to be today. In the case of Ben Carson, it was just his mother, but the Williams sisters were different, both their parents were tennis coaches, and their father had already started giving them tennis training since they were four and a half years old. Ben Carson, the first neurosurgeon to separate twins conjoined in the head, was initially a below-average student who never taught he could ever be better but his mother saw something different in him and made sure that he doesn't watch more than three television programs and read two books in a week which later turned out to be the solution, thanks to his mother, Ben Carson is one of the most successful doctors of all time.

- **Maintaining a good relationship with your kid.** This is very important because it is the determinant for all other things. Your kids won't learn and stick to what you teach them if you don't have a good and cordial relationship, so you need to ensure the presence of a strong relationship to achieve your parenting goals.

Also, a parent, if religious, builds the child according to the way of the religion, religious parents teach their children the ways of their religion, as a parent you ought to make sure your kids are sound both spiritually and physically. I believe that all the above-stated points have covered everything a parent aims to achieve pertaining to their kids.

What do you expect from your child?

Parents should basically expect nothing from their babies, initially, they are like empty containers or blank papers, that you are expected to fill up or write on, but as you are in your stage of zero-expectations, brace yourself for a series of events that occur as a result of cluelessness. So, you are to expect nothing and at the same time, a whole lot. Since babies are blank, empty, and don't know what is wrong or what is right, then you should expect a lot of "what is wrong." You now must help and guide them throughout this learning stage.

At this learning stage, kids display a lot of act that might want to piss you off, here are some:

- **Mouthing:** Babies generally do not know of any other way to examine and identify objects, so they just take everything they see and up it goes into the mouth. They don't understand texture by just touching or feeling the object, the object has to go into their mouth, it's only then they know whether it is edible or not, because, at this stage edible or inedible are the only two categories to which they classify objects they come across.

- **Smiling and Crying as the only means of communication:** At their tender age, when they haven't yet learned how to speak, these are the only two ways by which they express their feelings. Smiling, of course, is their way of showing happiness, an expression of satisfaction and excitement, crying, on the other hand, is how our toddlers try to make their feelings known when they are unhappy. Toddlers cry for numerous different reasons, which could include discomfort, hunger, being around unrecognized faces, et cetera. So, when babies start to cry, it is left to the parent to identify what is wrong and promptly take care of the situation.

- **Expect to have sleepless nights:** Babies have only one routine every day, which is to ESP (eat, sleep, and play). After sleeping a lot during the day, they tend to wake up at night, and when they wake up, that means your attention is needed, you have only two choices, to get up and attend to them or they disturb your sleep with loud, nonstop crying. Sometimes, they need food, water, need their diapers changed, and so on. Be sure to always be at their service.

- **Be ready for some things to get broken:** Throwing, smashing, beating, hitting ,et cetera, of things is fun to toddlers, and in the process of having fun, they get to destroy things that may be valuable, like perfume bottles, glass table, even some of their own toys, et cetera, you have to be very careful with what you leave around them, that way you can prevent and reduce the rate at which things get broken.

- **Tantrums and other modes of expressing dissatisfaction:** kids can display their anger in different ways, but the most common is usually tantrums. When you and your kids have disagreements, they want to show their dissatisfaction with the decision, other expressions of anger may include hard stomping, biting, hitting, kicking, et cetera.

Types of Parents

Researchers have stated that there are four types of parents: Authoritative, Permissive, Authoritarian, and Uninvolved. Authoritative is being perceived as the most reasonable and balanced of all other types, as they either have one problem or the other. In the cases of authoritarian and permissive, these two types are the extremes, the permissive is extremely lenient while the authoritarian is extremely controlling. However, the worst and most damaging type is the uninvolved. I will give a short explanation on each and how they can be exercised below.

The authoritative parent. This is the best method or type of parenting, the reason being that parents with this method are not overly harsh, neither are they extremely lenient. This is a mix of rules and freedom in which the kids are not subjected to only the will of the parents and at the same time know that there is a limit to how free they are. In this method, there are consequences for every wrong action, and there are rewards for, not all, but some positivity, your kid doesn't get a reward for eating, but you can sometimes reward your kid for some kind of display of obedience or any other thing you deem fit to be called a good deed, at least for a toddler, so as to make them keep the good deed up.

Authoritative parents:

- *Let their kids know what they expect from them; morally, academically.*

- *Set rules and regulations that have consequences if dishonored; well-planned daily schedule for important and basic things that have to be followed duly, although not when extremely uncomfortable, and backed with reasons and explanations.*

- *Create a chance for good and regular communication, which promotes a strong parent-child relationship.*

- *Are not afraid to implement consequences for kids' wrongdoings.*

- *Make sure to keep promises made to kids.*

This kind of parenting is the one that helps build kids' personalities, this mostly bears the fruit of self-confidence, self-belief, and high self-esteem.

The permissive parent. These are parents that allow "too much freedom" for their kids, they literally *spoil* their kids with a lot of consequence-free actions with the fear of not wanting to upset or offend their kids. This set of parents act more like "best friends" than parents. In permissive parenting, while showing a lot of love and affection towards kids, they tend to be overly lenient and delicate with them.

Permissive parents:

- *Show so much love and affection towards kids.*

- *Give the mammoth rewards for kids' minutest efforts.*

- *Always try to avoid kids' anger even if it requires not correcting them.*

- *Unlike the authoritative, have no rule or consequences and always willing to compromise even if there is any, so as not to tamper with their temper.*

This type of parenting, however, doesn't help in the building of the child's personality as it most times result in a lot of negatives like self-centeredness, very low socialization skills which make it hard for them to build and keep good relationships with people, kids brought up with this kind of method tend to become very saucy, and have no regard for authority.

The authoritarian parent. A type of parent with very high conditions and code of conduct, the authoritarian is similar to the authoritative, in the sense that they both set rules and principles but the difference is that the rules and regulations of the authoritative are detailed, but the authoritarian's are always overly strict and without any reasons or explanations. The authoritarian parents believe that children have no rights whatsoever to question their authority, once they say "go," it is "go," there is no "go because," "go so that," whatever they say is final!

Authoritarian parents:

- *Do not believe kids have a say; believe kids aren't to be heard, only to be seen.*

- *Give no reason for rules; they believe they have no reason to explain to their kids why rules and regulations are being set.*

- *Have no problem with using punishment as a means of discipline.*

- *Give their children little or no chance to make their own decisions or choices.*

- *Makes sure rules are obeyed no matter what.*

- *Don't give much time to a showing of affections and emotions.*

The authoritarian type of parenting has a really strong effect on the confidence and self-esteem of the kid. The fact that they are never given a chance to affect their self-assurance. Parents that find themselves in this category might want to try and be a little softer for the child's sake.

The neglectful or uninvolved parent. This is a very harmful type of parenting in where the parent has little or no involvement in the life of the kid. This actually is not very common as no responsible parent would want to neglect their children, but some parents actually think this method aids in making the children strong on their own. Causes of cases like this can include, having no clue on how to handle their children, not wanting to invade their child's privacy, having jobs that require a lot of their time and other numerous reasons.

Uninvolved parents:

- *Give little or no attention and spend less amount of time with their kids.*

- *Have not-very-close relationships with their kids.*

- *Less involvement in their kids' outside-home activities.*

This type is another type that can also affect the self-esteem of kids. Parents that find themselves in this category should do something about it, and try to adjust; if not, you might want to contact an expert for professional advice.

Some parents might find themselves exhibiting traits of more than one method, just be sure to choose the type that fits your kids, although the most advisable is the authoritarian parenting method.

Talking to toddlers

A bility to communicate with our toddlers in a way that they can understand is an asset that every parent should possess, although it might not be easy, it is possible through the help of some key information that I will be sharing with you shortly. You don't want to live the nightmare of having your toddlers get your message wrong or misinterpreted. There are ways by which you can be sure to establish a good communication with your kids, either when you're just talking to them or when the talk is for some discipline and correction. First, we discuss the approach to employ when talking to your kids, then we move onto the part where you implement discipline.

Tips on establishing good communication with toddlers

- **Speak normally:** You might be tricked into thinking that talking to your toddlers like they do makes them understand you better, no, in fact, it might even upset them, why? Because it might seem like you're trying to mock them. The truth is, what you call "baby language" is the best result of their effort to speak like we(adults) do. They are always eager to be able to do the things they see us do, but, like every person trying to learn something new, there is a slow beginning. Now, let me ask you this, as a person trying to learn how to play tennis, will you be pleased if your trainer drops the egg(ball) to bounce before hitting it with a bat instead serving normally? And say it's because he wants to come down your level and make it easy for you. That only reflects your incompetence, and does that not seem like mockery? You can only get better when you practice with people that are way better at it than you because that's how you discover and develop new skills and techniques, the same goes for the kids. Also, it's only hard for them to speak, it's not as hard for them to listen and hear. Although it is good to try to come to our babies' level for better understand, it can only be advised in some other aspects, not while talking.

Note: They can only learn from the original, not from the imitation of their own sub-standard version.

- **Keep it short and simple:** too many words will confuse your toddler, so, it is advised that you keep your information short and simple, for a quicker, easier understanding, but be careful not to misunderstand a toddler's "quicker" for an adult's. Excessive words can sound like gibberish to toddlers, Imagine, extracting a question from an engineering mathematics textbook for a second grader to do.

How to talk to toddlers when trying to discipline them

- **Talk with subtlety:** Nobody, not even toddlers, wants to be ordered around, so refrain from using a commanding voice. The mind is built in a way that it tends to defend itself against an imposing or enforcing authority, this makes the kid tend to refuse instructions that sound like orders. For example, instead of shouting, "Daniel! Stop bouncing on the couch", you could use, "Danny boy, mummy wants you to sit still on the couch" a little slowly, that gives a tone of subtlety. Don't ever Yell!

- **Find substitutes for NO!** Why do companies change their commercials from time to time? We get tired of what we are used to. When you always say no to your kids, they get used to it, thereby reducing the effect it has on them. Instead, try and erase that sense of negativity and replace it with some sense of positivity. For example, when trying to stop finger sucking, offer suckers, and say to them, "why don't you suck this instead, we don't want our fingers to get wet and smelly."

- **Avoid making threats:** It is naturally in human nature to want to dare, we like to see what comes after a threat has been made. Therefore, refrain from adding "or else" in your instructions, it calls out the inbuilt daring nature, thereby raising the tendency of refusal to comply.

- **Show seriousness:** Like adults, toddlers like to get involved when they recognize a level of seriousness. Toddlers too can be serious at times, even though they can be very playful with almost everything. For example, you want Diana to stop hitting the perfume bottle on the shelf, you don't just sit where you are and ask her to stop, rather, you get up, go closer and make your point known, the fact that you got up from where you were seating, shows a level of seriousness about that subject matter.

Setting Limits

L imit setting is another form of discipline for kids. It is very essential for parents to make it known to their kids that there are certain limits that shouldn't be crossed.

The primary purpose of setting limits is to help develop self-control and discipline for kids, but there are other reasons like protection of property, and protection of kids from physical harm. Limit setting helps significantly in the building of the child's personality. In a few lines, I'll discuss how limit setting helps in each of the above-stated purposes.

- **Self-control and discipline:** when kids have learned to control themselves and stay within the limits that have been set for them, it becomes a habit, and it sticks with them, the habit then rise whenever it is needed. It becomes part of them.

- **Protection of properties:** When kids learn to control themselves and put a limit to some of the unpleasant but fun giving modes of playing, they display, like smashing, hitting, beating, tearing, there will be a reduction in how they destroy our valuable properties.

- **Protection of kids from physical harm:** some of the injuries our toddlers have, are caused by themselves, but if the causes have been identified and limits have been set regarding them, when the rules are duly followed, then it will definitely put an end to kids injuring themselves.

***

When trying to set limits for your kids, you don't want to get it wrong so as to preserve its main purpose.

Tips for setting limits

- Be sure to set only reasonable limits; do not set limits that extreme.

- Set only important and necessary limits.

- State your rules clearly; make sure your kids understand.

- Be precise; make sure that your kids can relate a consequence to its offense.

- Be consistent; be sure not to fluctuate when implementing consequences.

- Never give in; even if the offense continues to occur.

Key to Toddler Cooperation

A lot of parents try but still find it hard to get their kids to cooperate in their endless day to day activities, do you find yourself having this problem? Well, you are not alone, there are many other parents out there with the same problem.

The main cause of this problem is misinterpretation and misunderstanding, even with adults, cooperation might be unattainable if there is a little misunderstanding, since it can happen between matured people, how much more a toddler who is yet to even have the knowledge of the basics of life.

Therefore, with what has been stated in the previous paragraph, it is safe to say the main keys to unlocking your toddler's cooperation are:

- *Good communication*

- *Better Understanding*

- *A warm and cordial parent-child relationship*

When all these are present between the child and the parent, then, cooperation is easily achieved. However, there are still some tips that are needed to get a kids' full cooperation:

- **Let your kids feel like they are in control:** Allowing your kids to make some of their own choices sometimes, erases the feeling that they are being controlled, that there is a superior and imposing authority and gives them the impression that they are in control, that way, they tend to give their full cooperation.

- **Always exercise patience:** You will need to have a lot of this when dealing with your kids, toddlers are not known for prompt responses, there might be some cases where you will be required to do some repetition, you might need to repeat things for better understanding for them.

- **Try finding something to praise about them:** Always try to praise every little good deed your kids do, every human feels happy when they are appreciated, the kids too are not left out, and when they get praised for doing something, they always want to do that same thing the more so that they'll get praised the more.

- **Make eye contacts:** Get their attention by making eye contacts, eye contacts bring emotional connections between parents and their kids.

- **Use the replacement method:** When you want to take something away from your kids to prevent them it from getting damaged, but they still want to keep playing with it, try replacing it with something else that can catch their attention too, then they can agree and cooperate with you on releasing the one you want to take away from them.

Toddler cooperation is not all about making them do what you want, it could require you to do some sacrificing. It's more about making peace reign, although, you are not advised to indulge them.

Give Your Toddler Choices and Gain Control

Giving toddlers choices is a measure employed to gain cooperation and to maintain good behavior in kids. When you want your kids to do something, and you know you're going to have a difficult time getting them to do so, you find some allowable choice to give to them, meanwhile stating the main reason behind the situation, the choices you give them distracts them from the original motive, for example, it's bedtime, and you want to ask your kid to go to bed, you know she is not ready to but she has to, you just go, "Maddy, it's time for bed, do you want your pajamas or your nightgown?" That way, she just focuses on choosing one of the two, and she goes to bed, problem solved. That's what I call "having the situation under control."

Importance of giving choices

- **They learn all about consequences of choices:** When making choices, children get to

33

know that actions have consequences (consequences aren't necessarily negative), they get to know, so it helps them in future decision-making situations.

- **Makes them feel respected:** When you let your kids choose for themselves, and you respect their opinion, this shows that you actually respect them. It pleases them to know that they are acknowledged thereby multiply your chances of getting their cooperation.

- **Satisfies their urge for power and control:** Kids naturally want to feel independent and believe they can do things on their own, by allowing them to make their own choices, you have ultimately satisfied that urge.

- **Attracts their cooperation:** Choice offering is one of the main and important measures employed when trying to gain the cooperation of toddlers.

When Gentle Discipline is Not Enough

With all that has been discussed, we can tell that aggressive discipline is not welcome, but when nonaggressive discipline in not working, is it ok to use to aggressive measures? When we have tried every possible way to correct kids, but they are not heeding, it's only normal to think towards aggressiveness, but it's never right to employ methods that can harm the kids (physically, mentally, and emotionally).

Kids like this are called different names by different people, but the most popular is Strong-willed. Strong-willed kids are kids that stand by what they believe, no matter what you do to try to change them, you can't force a change out them, except if they are willing to. When strong-willed kids say "NO," it means no.

Some characteristics of strong-willed kids

Strong-willed kids show some characteristics that other kids don't,

- **Can be very persistent:** Strong-willed kids never give in, they enjoy power-struggling and battle for supremacy, and it is very convenient for them to argue for a very long time, there will going and going. They also always want to get what they think they deserve or desire.

- **Question authority:** These kids don't just accept whatever you tell them, they always want you to give them reasons. They always demand to know why they should do whatever you ask them to.

- **Deep and frequent outbursts:** Spirited kids, as they are also called, are quick to display their anger, tantrums in strong willed kids are stronger, they can go extreme and do things like foot-stomping, throwing themselves, very loud yelling, et cetera, at the floor, in a bid to make their feelings (of anger) known.

- **Can't wait, impatient, but hate to be rushed:** They are very bad at being patient, they hate to wait for something for too long, but the funny irony is that when it comes to them, they like to work at their pace, they never want to be rushed.

- **They like dominance:** They like to dominate and behave in a bossy kind of way; they always want to be in control.

- **Don't care about rules:** They live by their own rules alone; they like to decide for themselves.

Spirited kids have a bright side to them in the sense that if well guided, which is tough to do because of their independent mentality, they grow up to have very strong personalities comprised of a very high self-esteem, very strong self-confident, high problem-solving skills due to their independent mentality, never give up spirit and leadership ability.

Dealing with Strong-Willed Toddlers

The following are the general tips in dealing with your toddlers. Different situations require different solutions, it is now your duty as a parent to identify what works for your kids.

- **Acknowledge their feeling:** Show them that you understand their feelings and reason for their outburst, that will calm them down.

- **Identify what triggers their anger:** You have to try to identify regular causes for their anger, then try avoiding the "avoidable" ones, be careful not to indulge them, do not avoid corrective measures, only things that are avoidable should be avoided.

- **Always follow through:** When rules are broken, or limits are crossed, be sure to follow through with consequences.

- **Give rewards for good behavior:** they will repeat good behaviors when rewarded until it becomes part of them.

- **Give timeouts:** It gives them time to calm down.

- **Stay calm:** Parents too have to work on themselves, sometimes we let our anger affect our actions, we have to stay calm.

All other previously stated measures will work on strong-willed children but needs extra work, just stay calm and keep trying, and you will find that patience yields result.

Lead by Your Deeds

With your kids, you are not just a parent, you are also a leader and role model. Now, as a leader, you are expected to teach your kids values that make a human being, as a leader, you are expected to guide them through your teachings, and as a role model, you are expected to show what you teach. Be sure to lead your kids by example, setting good examples helps shape the lives of kids as their brain tends to stick with what they have learned as infants, reflections of parents' behavior can be seen on their kids because kids unconsciously emulate their parent's behavior.

"Do as I say" is very common with parents, it easily lets your child know that having tantrums and outbursts is bad, but it's bad when you can't even seem to control yourself, you flare up at any little misunderstanding, you are confusing the child, if you are going to give your children some training, then you should be ready to learn too, you will also have to make some sacrifices, like the rate at which you used to drink, will have to be reduced to the barest minimum so as not to give the child a wrong perception on drinking, how your child views drinking depends on what they see you do. You can't be a drunk and expect your kids to have the idea "drink responsibly," that will give the feeling that it's a normal way of life.

"Do as I do" is, however, recommended. It might require drastic reduction or complete stoppage of old habits, as they might confuse kids on what to believe, the danger of not leading by example is that, kids tend to choose what you showcase over what you tell them, thereby making them more likely to emulate the negative habits over the more acceptable ones you are trying to preach. Some parents believe they are who they are already but they just don't want their kids to do the same, thinking "this is me already, I don't think I can change anymore at the stage I'm in now, I just need to make sure my kids follow the right path and don't turn out like me, well, No! It's never too late for you to stop those habits you don't want your kids to emulate, even if you don't have a reason to stop them, do it for your kids if you think they're worth it.

Another advantage of showing and not just telling is that it might even change the minds of unheeding kids. When your kids that won't heed or cooperate notices the way you do things you say, they might want to change their minds and start to "do as you say and do."

Kids' relationship with other people is influenced by the way they see you interact with other people in every day to day activities.

Kids can also help us become better people if we are willing. Training our kids gives us a sense of responsibility, that sense of responsibility gives our lives purpose and meaning.

It is very essential to not only tell but show our kids how it is done. It is never too late for you or never too early for your kids, remember their brain holds on to what it has learned at a very tender age.

Part Two
Handling Everyday Situations

Going to Bed

Getting your toddler to bed sometimes is like single-handedly going to free hostages in a terrorist territory, it can be really tedious. After the whole stress-filled day, this is the one last war you have to fight every day, except the sleep comes naturally, going to bed for kids sounds like a punishment, why do I have to force my eyes to close? I am still very much active, that is what always goes on in their head each time you tell them, "it's time to go to bed."

How long do they need to sleep?

The number of hours kids need to sleep in a day changes with age, as they grow, the required length reduces. Kids at age one and two require eleven to fourteen hours while kids within the range of three to five require a lesser ten to thirteen hours of night sleep. Not only do they have a standard time for night sleep, they also have a stipulated amount of nap time, kids between one to two and half years need about two naps (usually one to three hours) a day, while for kids between two-and-a-half and five years, needs just one nap time (also about one to three hours long), mind you, naps too close to normal bedtime can cause sleepless nights for toddlers, so, be sure to set their nap time far from their night sleep, say for the ones that need two naptimes, the first could come around 11am through to 1pm and second around 3.30pm through to 5pm, that way it easier to make them sleep at night, that when they wake from nap at around 6.30pm or 7pm. Kids that fail to observe naptime should be made to have some quiet time to give them some rest, it can serve as a close substitute to a nap.

However, as much as we know our kids need this sleep for proper growth and development, they don't know about that, that is why they make us climb the Everest each time we try to put them to sleep. Here are some ways by which our "putting to bed" struggles can be overcome.

Tips on putting toddlers to bed

There are certain measures that can be taken to really overcome the struggles of putting toddlers to sleep.

- **Calm and quiet pre-bedtime:** The few hours to bedtime should be quiet and stress-free in order to prevent them from being overly active, which could make it harder for them to sleep.

- **Set a consistent daily nighttime routine:** Make your toddler get used to a daily routine that occurs immediately before their bedtime. When this routine is repeated every night and what comes next is sleep, the kid is then going to expect this routine every night, knowing that after all, it will end with him/ her asleep. Bedtime routine can include teeth-brushing and bathing, putting on pajamas, storybook reading, and rocking accompanied by a lullaby, routine should be carried out in this exact order. Some toddlers might not like night baths, and as this might cause some fight back, which could make them active, we could just probably skip this part. Also, some times, the goal might have been accomplished while reading the bedtime story, thereby leaving the lullaby needless, but if the kid hasn't slept after the story reading, singing the lullaby might not work at once, but repeated singing should do the trick. Be sure to add a goodnight kiss after they have fallen asleep.

- **Avoid power struggles by offering choices:** Gain power by giving power to toddler, when he is made to control what happens, then, he is happy to do what he has chosen. In the case of putting on the pajamas as mentioned in the previous point, you present two pajamas and ask him to decide which one he wants, you could also ask when it's bath time if he wants to brush his teeth before or after a bath. Doing this and following the routine definitely makes it easier for them to sleep.

- **Dim lights:** Except in the case of fear, where your kids are scared of the dark (which usually only begins when they are older toddlers), it's easier to sleep in the presence of lesser light.

- **Provide a snuggly sleeping environment:** Your toddler should sleep in a cozy and comfortable place, a clean and well-laid bed in a beautiful and appealing environment. A colorful and decorated bed area is likely to attract toddlers and give them some sort of satisfaction.

- **Balanced daytime exercise and rest:** Ensure that your toddler has enough exercise or activity as well as enough rest during the day, it aids their mental balance and keeps their body in a perfect working condition, this is another essential element in helping them get a sound sleep.

However, it is important to know that as toddlers grow, they need to learn how to sleep off on their own. That can be achieved by leaving them to do so. So, after the nighttime routine, instead of rocking to sleep, you could just rock the baby half-way (almost but not yet asleep) and leave her to sleep on her own, mind you, this might seem impossible at first,(since the kid, has got used to being rocked to sleep) she might begin to cry when she discovers your absence, just keep repeating this, she'll get used to it.

Tidiness of the Room

Having tidy kids can sound really impossible, but trust me, it is achievable. The truth is, kids can't be expected to be perfect, but it is possible to get a reasonable level of tidiness in kids. This is a very important habit to inculcate in a child, and it is not too early if it started while they are still very young, because what they learn at a very tender age is what they will grow up with. Getting your older kids to keep their room tidy is equal to rock-climbing, let alone your toddlers. While very little kids of ages between a year and two are not really expected to do much, toddlers from three can be given a couple of lessons on room tidiness. Wondering how this can be pulled off? Check out these tips below.

Tips on how to encourage toddlers' room tidiness.

- **Practice what you teach:** First of all, if you want to encourage your toddler to be tidy and keep their room tidy, you have to show them what you want to teach them. Although our toddlers can't be as perfect as we are, they still want to try and make a photocopy of the things they see us do.

- **Create a particular place for every single thing in their room:** Seeing us do these things is not enough, toddlers will still need our help in the arrangement of the things in their room. Having a space for everything makes it easier for them to keep their room tidy because they won't get confused as to where to put and keep each object. We can also help them further with arrangements by using labels, put a label on each object and a matching one in the place designated for it. For example, you can label the toy box and put a matching label in the space you have created for it in the cabinet. You can also try getting room furniture that doubles as equipment for the organization.

- **Let them know:** Oral explanation should also be employed; constant repetition might be required as toddlers would need a lot of reminding. Also, let them know that untidiness is not acceptable and can't be allowed.

- **A consistently seen reminder:** Apart from the oral reminder, a visual reminder like a picture of how their room is supposed to look like should be placed in their room, this will help them remember each time they see it.

- **Encourage self-discipline:** Your kids should know how to pick up after themselves, even when you're not there. Picking things up immediately and putting them in place will help reduce littering so that there won't be much work cleaning the room.

- **Do away with useless things:** Free up spaces in the room by getting rid of any and every unneeded object, this helps by making arrangements and placing of things easy, as there will be lesser things to arrange.

- **Give them a say:** In deciding and designating places for things in the room, giving them a chance to be part of the decision process will make them want to follow through since the decision was also made by them. Also allow them a say while arranging the room, ask them, where should we hang the shelf, here or there?

- **Appreciate good deeds:** Good deeds should earn kids your praises, it urges them to want to do more.

Your toddlers are not expected to do all the chores even though it's their room, in fact, they are just to do only a tiny little bit in everything, the idea is just to promote tidy habits and reduce the workload on parents as their room won't need much effort after the kids have been taught to maintain a level of tidiness.

Mouthing Everything

Toddlers are known for directing every object they come across, into their mouths, at some point in their toddlerness, that is because they have no other method of identifying an object, their mouth is their only means of exploring their immediate environment as this is the main reason for mouthing. The stage of teething can also be a cause for toddlers mouthing stuff, from their blankets, to your mobile phones, to their toys and so on, when kids are going through the teething process, they derive some soothing relief from biting and chewing objects that they find around them. As a parent, this might bother you as it is not appealing hygiene wise, but you don't have to let it, because mouthing is a natural occurrence in the growth and development of toddlers, you only have to be careful of the things you leave around them, so as to avoid them taking in substances that can cause harm to their health, be sure to keep toxic substances and inedible objects that are small enough to be swallowed out of their reach, and make sure that "out of their reach" is not a climbable place, because toddlers can be good with climbing at times. Additionally, if you are the type that doesn't feel too good about your kids putting just about everything in their mouth then you should probably get teethers, you would feel a little more comfortable when you know what they are chewing is something that has been designed to be chewed, mind you, you have to be careful with the type of teethers you get, there are some that can contain chemicals, personally, I'll recommend that you get uncoated wooden ones, since plastic or silicone can't be fully trusted.

However, as much as oral mouthing is necessary and inevitable, it has a certain time for which it should run, it is supposed to occur when the kid is between one and two years old, if a kid still keeps mouthing six months later, then there is a possibility of an oral fixation. Oral fixation is when a baby can't stop putting things into the mouth, even after passing the mouthing stage. If the kid continues with oral fixation, you will have to consult a professional (pediatrician).

Table Manners and Eating Habits

Have you ever heard of any more contrasting words than "kids and table manners"? Chances are very slim, but as contrasting as they can be, there are corrections that can be made to allow for the replacement of contrast with compatibility. Table manners, like other good manners, can be very hard to teach to toddlers, but it is important to know that it is a gradual process, which could take a really long time to manifest. It is also not wrong to start these teachings at a very early stage as many parents might think, the truth, actually, is to begin to teach them these manners at that very early stage, say when they are about a year old, at the initial stage (that time they are about a year old), your efforts might appear futile, but you have to trust that with time it becomes fruitful, and by the time they get to three, you should start to see some improvements. Table manners in toddlers is not all about just the etiquettes (how to hold and use your fork and knife, how to place your napkin, sitting posture, etc.), while table manners in toddlers contains all that, it also involves stopping some of those general toddler eating habits (like throwing of food all over the place, mashing, spitting of already mouthed food, and all others). I will discuss with you shortly ways you can curb their unacceptable eating habits, but before that, I will give a list of the general table manners everyone needs to inculcate and exhibit. Teach your kids

- To wash their hands before coming to the table.

- To place napkins on their laps before eating commences.

- To sit upright and be sure to keep elbows off the table.

- To wait until everyone is seated, settled, and served before starting to eat.

- Never to talk with food in mouth, and to keep the mouth closed while chewing.

- Ask to be handed whatever is out of reach, with politeness, and the use of the word "please," followed with a "thank you."

- To never complain about what has been served, a show of politeness is required in the case of a medical condition or recommendation that states foods that shouldn't be eaten.

- How to properly handle and use cutlery.

- To never yell, shout, or make other improper, irritating, rude or disturbing noises like slurping and others, at the table.

- To always use the polite words, "please, and thank you."

- To never make use of phones or other electronic devices (iPads, iPods, games, etc.) while at the table.

- To never get up from the table until everyone at the table is finished, while there might be a good reason to leave, you should at least ask to be excused.

- And last but not least, always say "thank you" to show appreciation after a meal, and be sure to offer help in clearing the table.

As much as all these lessons are essential, they can't all be taught at the same time or at any time, there are a lot of these that would be too complicated for the understanding of toddlers, so they are best kept for later years when the kids can totally understand what they are being taught.

While all these are the general etiquette to be taught and shown, toddlers still exhibit some unacceptable habits that parents need to find a way to curb. When kids start displaying their creativity in food artistry, parents have the job of making them know that their actions are unacceptable, but this shouldn't be done by yelling or fuss making, you have to be calm as kids need a lot of reminding before they can fully take in the lessons you are giving. Also, doing some things for them consistently will help them know that, that is the way of life, for example, always wash their hands and face before coming to the table, they will eventually understand that that's what they are supposed to do, don't be surprised when you see them going to do so when it's meal time, although, you might need to do it properly, at least, they're getting the message. Another scenario is when you give your toddlers about four slices or pieces of whatever it is, and they start throwing and flinging all over the place, you can start by reducing the slices to one, when the food in question is liquid, you can take it away for a little while and then return, if he starts spilling again, take it again and over and over again, she will then know that, you are taking it away because she is spilling, she gets the message and will then know it is bad to spill or throw food. You should also be sure to communicate with them, tell them what and what is not acceptable, but softly and calmly.

Also, kids learn from what they see, so be sure to behave the way you want them to, at the table (and everywhere) because they'll want to copy you. They want to do the things you do.

Gadgets and TV

It's no news that kids nowadays are born with in-built manuals for electronic devices and gadgets in their brains. Toddlers are attracted to any thing that has a screen, but these screens, however, according to research, although they have their benefits, have been found to do more harm than good, therefore, parents are warned to put a limit on the amount of time their kids spend on screens (TVs, video games, iPads or tabs, phones, and every other thing that has a screen). Babies in the age range of 0-18 months, advisably, are not allowed any form of screen (except, maybe it's as important as videos chatting with family and friends-which actually helps in enhancing good communication skills). As they grow, they are allowed to use screens, bigger toddlers are allowed more time than more little ones, but the general maximum amount of screen time allowed for a toddler is One hour. Some parents need some space sometimes from their kids, like when they want to cook in peace or a little chat with their partner or some other important talk, so they just buy themselves some time by giving their kids the chance to use a screened device and do not care if the standard limit has been exceeded, Wrong, fine you need some time but you kid is not helping, you still don't have to make that your last resort.

Screen time for toddlers:

0 - 18 months: no screen time (except for video chatting)

18 - 24 months: some screen time with parental guidance

2 - 5 years: a maximum of one hour a day (also with some parental guidance)

Disadvantage of screen time

As much entertainment and enjoyment kids derive from these devices, spending too much time with them can cause some problems in the development of kids. When kids spend too much time with these screens, they have no time for some real-life developmental activities in the sense that, they have lesser time to practice walking, they have lesser time for interactions which is supposed to build their communication skills and abilities. Too much time on screens can cause for a sedentary lifestyle, which in turn increases chances for obesity.

Therefore, the two major disadvantages of excessive screen time are:

- *Setbacks in kid's development*

- *Sedentary lifestyle that eventually causes Obesity.*

Tips on handling toddlers' gadgets and TV

- **Set a daily schedule.** A daily schedule has to be set in order to limit the screen time of your toddlers, a daily schedule that has a lot of non-screen time. Be sure to fix in other exciting, entertaining, and of course, occupying activities so as to keep them busy, and stop them from believing that screens are the only option available in whiling away the time.

- **Give explanations.** Use your words, to let your kids know that too much time on screens can cause harm to their health, give them reasons why they can't watch the TV, or play their videos games, or watch Netflix.

- **Parental guidance.** Your presence at screen time is very important, be with your kids at screen time so that you can guide them through what they are watching (or playing). This also creates a chance for interactions thereby building their communication skills.

- **Only recommendable apps and games.** In the case of apps and games, be sure that the apps you get for them are tested, trusted and recommended ones, that not only entertains but also educates. In other words, make their time spent in front of TV or any app worthwhile.

- **Parental control.** Be sure to make use of the parental control systems that are provided in TVs, phones, and other gadgets, in case of any form of absence.

Helping Parents

When we think "toddlers," what comes after is "play," especially when we are busy, maybe doing some house chore or the other, we never believe our toddlers can be of help. Parents need to learn to understand their kids (even though it's easier to say than to execute), we also need to understand that toddlers too, apart from tantrums and other displays of anger, can be serious at times. When they see us doing some things, they also want to try, but parents always think otherwise. Sometimes, when we even recognize their willingness to help, we simply refuse and tell them "no, you'll get to help when you're bigger." We also just prefer to do these things by ourselves just because, if we allow them to do it, they end up messing it up, it is true toddlers aren't yet perfect at doing these things, but stopping them from trying doesn't help either. Allowing kids to help in house chores aids in their growth and development into adults.

Benefits

Below are some good returns of allowing toddlers to help with tasks.

- **Sense of belonging:** When kids get involved in doing the household chores, they get the feeling that they, too, are recognized as an important part of the family.

- **Confidence builder:** Being allowed to a part in the house chores make them know that you have trust in their abilities (no matter how tiny it might seem), this, therefore, gives them a level of confidence which eventually becomes part and parcel of their personality.

- **Enhances their cooperation with others:** Working together with your toddlers in doing house chores help build their collaboration and cooperation skills. Working with other people won't be hard for them since it's what they've been doing since toddler-age.

- **Promotes appreciative spirit:** When kids get appreciated for helping, they grow to become appreciative beings, since you are their role model.

- **Builds self-discipline:** Self-discipline and responsibility taking are also portrayed by kids who are involved in carrying out house chores.

However, with all these being listed, it's not all kids that want to help at all time, and getting them involved when they are not interested initially can be exhausting, but they can be left alone because toddlers need to be taught to help with house chores for their personality's sake, so some tips have been developed in order to get them to help.

Tips for getting toddlers to help

- **Not by force:** As I have always said, kids, like adults, never like being bossed around or dictated to, there is no room for dictatorship if you want to get them to help out with house chores or other things, let them decide they want to, when they are forced, there is a very high tendency for refusal.

- **Encourage collaborative work:** Do not make tasks like clothes folding personal, instead of asking them to fold their own clothes while you fold yours, you can just allow them to fold anyone.

- **Expect and allow the mess.** It is true that help from toddlers can make things a little slower, sloppier and messy, but you have to learn to allow for the mess to happen, although you will take care of it, it shouldn't be immediately, so as to not give your kid the wrong impression.

- **No task is too small:** Be sure to expose your kid to every possible chore, give a wide range of tasks from helping while sweeping, to helping out in the garden, to helping with laundry and dishes. Do not limit their exploration, try and make them redirect their energy usage from throwing things, hitting, and all that show of power, into using it for useful work for the family.

- **Sense of contribution:** The chores you let them do, of course, can't be "big," but be sure that the tiny ones they do are significantly important that it gives them the impression that they are truly contributing.

Kids also develop gross and fine motor skills when they carry out certain tasks (with parents' help, of course), involvement in chores also help sharpen Kids' brain, which helps improve their problem-solving skills.

Fights Over the Table

Your toddler frequently gives you a hard time each meal time, this can happen as a result of a variety of reasons. Below is a list of possible causes of toddlers' mealtime fight and their respective solutions.

- **You show too much attention.** When you concentrate too much on your kid at mealtime; showing too much concern about how much they eat, showing excitement when they eat well, or displeasure when they eat less. It puts pressure on them, which displeases them, and in turn, they lose interest, then the war begins.

  You can give them some amount of freedom and a sense of independence at mealtime. When they feel they are in control, then they don't get to feel that eating is an obligation.

- **Transition problem.** They find it hard to transit from the previous or present activities to mealtime. When kids are busy with something else right before mealtime, any attempt to make them leave what they are doing to come to the table will be met with a stiff refusal.

You have to work the transition into them before time, notifying them beforehand is essential so that when the time finally comes, they will be prepared. For example, when it's about ten minutes before mealtime, you say to them, "Amber, you have eight minutes until mealtime, you'll need the two minutes extra time.

- **Tiredness.** Kids, after so much unrest, become too tired to do anything, and yes, they can also be too tired to eat.

  Be sure to plan your kids daily schedule well, with a balanced amount of rest and activity so that they don't eventually become over-worked or stressed out.

- **Snack, eaten too close to mealtime.** When your kid has a satisfying snack too close to mealtime, he becomes filled up, and digestion has not yet fully taken place when it is time for meal, he, of course, would refuse to eat.

Be sure to give snacks further from mealtime, there should be at least two hours interval between the snack and mealtimes.

- **Taste disorders.** Your kid might be having a condition of taste disorder, which can change how some foods taste. A specialist (pediatrician) should be consulted ASAP.

Public Tantrums

As gentle-souled as kids are, they get angry too (actually, a lot), and they don't hesitate to show their displeasure at all. Kids are very plain, when they're happy, you'll know, and when it's the otherwise, they won't fail in showing you that either. Now, kids don't know where or where not to show their other side, be it at home, or in the bank, or in the white house with the press, if they feel displeasure, they will show it at once, they are not ready to wait till you get home before they sit you down and let you know. They do not know if they are making you feel embarrassed when they display tantrums in public places, but as parents, we always find a way to avoid these situations, although success might not be assured. Well, parents, here are few tips on how you can prevent or avoid your toddlers' public tantrums.

- **Clear your head:** First of all, you have to clear your head and free yourself from getting tricked into believing that toddlers plan to embarrass you in public with their tantrums. Toddlers just want to express themselves, and the only way they can show their anger is through tantrums.

- **Discover what causes problems:** Try and discover potential tantrum triggers, when you have done that, then you can try and avoid things like that, in the process, nullifying any possibility of tantrums. Some things that can trigger tantrums in toddlers can include hunger, tiredness, when they don't get what they want, a sudden change in the normal schedule, discomfort and so much more, in fact, there's nothing a toddler can't display tantrums for.

- **Full attention:** Be sure to always give your kids full attention every time, you must not get tired of doing that as they will need a lot of this at this stage of their life.

- **Always give them a chance to choose and decide:** Although there are times, we have to make the decisions for our kids, please do not hesitate at every chance you get to allow them to make their own choices. Who refuses his own decision or choice, you can only refuse when the choice was not made by you? When you are always choosing for them, it could trigger tantrums since it's a way of showing refusal.

- **Before-hand notice of what to expect:** To be forewarned is to be forearmed, when you give them a forenotice of how and what to do at a given time, they already know what to expect, so there is a lesser chance of the occurrence of tantrums. Mind you, a million times repetition might be needed because they really get your message.

However, no matter how much we try to prevent or avoid tantrums, toddlers will still be toddlers, so we still need to know the cure in case the prevention is not effective.

How to deal with public tantrums

The following are a few ways by which we can face or deal with toddlers' public tantrums.

- **Be calm:** Even in the middle of the great storm of your toddler's tantrum, you have to learn how to stay calm and keep your cool, aggressive measures like yelling, spanking and co. is never an option, it will only escalate the whole situation to the point that you won't even be able to handle the child's tantrum.

- **Deflection for distraction:** When you notice the imminence of a tantrum, you employ a medium of distraction that can help deflect their mind and turn the enraged mind into a jolly one. Draw their attention with something awkward and funny (probably a fart), this has already done pacifying that might have been needed three times more if the tantrum had taken over.

- **Show that you understand:** Showing that you understand their feelings and why they might be angry can help calm them down. Show them that you understand and be sure to explain to them the reason for whatever is the bone of contention.

- **Ignorance:** Sometimes, this is needed as the kid might be proving too stubborn and does not want to be dealt with gentle. This is about the highest form of aggressive approach that can be used in dealing with toddlers' public show of tantrums. You try to pretend as if you can't even hear the toddler screaming, after some time, the toddler eventually tires out and stops.

- **Never give in:** While you are trying to stop your toddler's tantrum, you still have to be careful to not always let her have her way, when you always grant a toddler's wish because of a display of tantrum, you are empowering the kid and making him believe tantrums will always get things done.

Monsters Under the Bed

Over the years, monsters under the bed has become one general fear for kids, kids are afraid of the dark because they can't see clearly and would probably be thinking "anything could be lurking in the dark", their brains even go to the extent of conjuring some scary monster figure in that darkness, this makes them feel unsafe and unprotected. It all still comes back to the parents; it is now our job to protect them and make them feel safe even if we know there are no such things as monsters lurking. The funny thing is that only older toddlers have this phobia, very little ones have nothing to worry about, just make sure they fall asleep, and they see you in the morning. This is actually a simple task for a parent, but the deal is, you have some playing-along to do.

First of all, you have to always check under their beds in their presence (you should let them see with their eyes too and make sure that there are no monsters under there. You also have to throw some assuring displays, for example, you can get any random thing (it could even be a white piece of cloth) and make them believe that as long as they have it hung over their head or at their room entrance, the monsters can never come close. You could also try leaving their room lights on so as to get rid of darkness, in case a bright light bulb won't let them sleep, you can just do them the favor of keeping it dim, you just need to have some form of light in the room, since darkness is the main cause.

It is understandable that you are tempted to tell them there is no such thing as monsters, but you don't have to do that because they would never fully agree with you, you're just gonna have to be patient until they outgrow that fear. It doesn't last forever.

Toilet Training

At some point, the use of diapers definitely will have to be stopped, although, not completely, toddlers might still have to wear diapers at times (mostly when going out). Parents wonder, "at what point or age should toilet training (can also be referred to as "potty training") be introduced?" there is actually no particular age for this, but it is known to usually happen when toddlers are between the ages of eighteen months and four years. Times and ages of readiness vary in different kids, parents have to be able to know when their toddlers are ready to stop using diapers, it's not like your toddler's going to come to you and say "Hey, I think I won't be needing a nappy anymore." Toddlers can be said to be ready:

- *When they can hold (time-length for holding increases gradually)*

- *If they can walk by themselves to the toilet*

- *When they can understand what you tell them*

- *When they can pull down without your help*

- *If they can let you know when they are pressed*

When you as a parent notice these, then you have the green light to take the diapers away. However, toddlers already showing signs doesn't mean they automatically know how to go about using the potty or toilet, there is still some tip you need to know in order to be able to introduce an effective training.

Tips on toilet-training toddlers

- **Patience:** You'll need a lot of this, as the operating speed of toddlers is relatively very low, you don't have to rush the process because it will take a really long time for them to digest everything and put them into practice. Just be calm and don't be pushed to apply force if there's a slow response or progress. A lot of repetition and reminding will also be needed.

- **Introduce the medium:** This involves bringing them in contact with the medium they are about to start using, place the potty (in the case of potty) where it's supposed to be and get them to see it, and then explain how they use it to them. If you are using a toilet, begin taking them to the toilet whenever you notice any sign of pressure (squirming, holding of genitals, showing of discomfort), place a box or stool to make it easy for them to sit, they can't sit comfortably when there is nothing for them to put their feet on. You can also do good to place attractive items in form of their favorite stickers, that can attract them and make them want to come back, it boosts their interest in using the toilet. Be also sure that they really understand what you have explained to them.

- **Quick response:** When you notice any signs of pressure, make sure to be quick to attend to them and take them where they are supposed to go, this helps relate the feeling to the action, when this is a constant action that follows the sensation, they then know that is what they are supposed to do.

- **Set out time for toilet use:** Set a schedule with a time interval (say two hours) for them to go and use the toilet, with your supervision. You can let them have something that'll keep them busy.

- **Teach them the after potty musts:** For hygiene's sake, they have to learn to wash thoroughly and properly after pooping or peeing.

- **Show only appreciation:** You should only show appreciation when they have done well, be careful not to give material rewards though as this will only mean you're indulging them, next time they won't do it if there is no reward, praising is rewarding enough for them. Also, be sure not to show your displeasure when there is a mistake as it is only normal and can kill their interest, you don't do all that when they were using diapers, so this might want to make them prefer using the nappy.

- **Don't be caught unprepared:** There would still be some imperfections at times, so you should have some replacements ready when outdoors in case of an emergency.

It's easier for kids to learn how to stay dry at day than at night, kids who already have toilet training in the day may still wet the bed at night although pooping at night is uncommon after age two. Protective measures like a waterproof cover might be needed for the bed to prevent it from getting wet. Boys can learn to pee while sitting first, and then learn to stand when after mastering bowel usage.

Teeth Care

Oral health care plays an important role when it comes to the health of a child, it is important to care for our toddlers' teeth as much as we care for every other part of the body. Why do I have to be really concerned about those temporary baby teeth? They're going to fall out anyway. Well, Tooth decay, caused by presence of bacteria on or around the tooth, this bacteria is caused by sugary edibles, causes discomfort for kids, also causes loss of tooth, these baby teeth lay the foundation for the formation of the permanent teeth, so, unhealthy milk teeth can affect the formation of the permanent teeth. Parents might believe that they don't have to care too much about their babies teeth when no actual teeth are present, but I'll have you know that babies actually already have teeth formed before birth, and at birth, babies already have 20 teeth hidden in the gum, and besides, in the absence of teeth, the gum is equally supposed to be seriously cared for.

Brushing

When cleaning the gum (before the first tooth comes out), a clean damp piece of cloth should be used to wipe the surface of the gums, then rinse the mouth with water. This clears away the bacteria and keeps the mouth clean.

When they start growing teeth, then you should begin using infant toothbrushes, very tiny size of fluoride-containing toothpaste can be used. The fluoride helps in the reduction of tooth decay.

When your child gets to about two-and-a-half years, you can start using a pea-sized amount of fluoride-containing toothpaste. You can allow them to hold the brush with you to get their cooperation as it might make them feel in control. Your kids will still need your supervision while brushing until they are about 9 - 10 years of age. Brushing should be done twice daily, in the morning and at night before bedtime.

Flossing

This should be done as soon the child's teeth begin touching each other. Flossing is advisably done right after brushing.

Procedure for brushing a toddler's teeth

Stay behind with the chin cupped in your hand, and head resting on your body, try brushing in front of a mirror. Clean the inside and outside of the gums and teeth by gently moving brush in circles around them (mind you, electric brushes don't require circular movement, just hold still and guide your hand through the teething), try lifting the lips to create space and allow for the proper penetration of the brush, angle the brush towards the gums. The chewing teeth should be thoroughly brushed by moving the brush back and forth, then gently brush the tongue to prevent mouth odor. Be sure to ask your kid to spit out to prevent swallowing of toothpaste, there isn't any need for rinsing because the fluoride left back can help strengthen the enamel and prevent tooth decay and cavity.

Brushing toddler's teeth might be made uneasy by them because it can be uncomfortable for them, you'll need to have a lot of patience and calmness.

- *Try getting more than one brush and toothpaste so they can get to choose and feel in control, in order to avoid a power struggle.*

- *Avoid using a hard brush.*

- *Start by following their lead and gently take over.*

- *Make brushing fun by adding some playfulness, you can even put the paste on the nose and be funny.*

- *Employ professional intervention by asking the dentist to explain to them why brushing is important, you can just remind them of that every time they want to refuse.*

Seeing the dentist is also very important, toddlers can start seeing the dentist within the first six months of the first tooth appearance, but if there is slow growth, they should start after their first twelve months.

Fights with Siblings

Siblings fighting with each other is another day-to-day experience a parent should expect. Fights can happen for literally any reason at all, kids can fight over toys, kids can fight for space, fights can even occur over who sits on daddy's lap, whatever it is, kids can fight over it.

Fights, sometimes, can be intentionally sparked by one child or the other, children can seek attention by any means possible, even if it is negative, after all, half bread is better than none. Competition is another reason why siblings fight each other, fights can happen over who does what first, first to have a bath, who gets dressed first, until the end of the world, kids will compete and fight for supremacy. In the twinkle of an eye, playtime can turn into wartime between siblings.

Having a younger sibling can be frustrating for a toddler, which would cause them to express their anger by trying to start a fight. A toddler is yet to understand what it means to have a younger one, all he knows is that one new little creature has come to hijack all the attention, love, and care he's been getting.

It's not an easy job for a parent who, by the addition of a new member into the family, now has to add refereeing to the long list of parental tasks. In fact, some parents find it hard to the extent that they never even know what to do when the war begins, this war which happens, at least, about six times a day. The following are some tips that should be taken for the tackling and reduction of the daily inevitable sibling squabbles.

- **Kids learn from what they see:** Make sure you are not just telling your kids to do as you say, behave how you want them to copy, when your kids see that you handle everything that comes your way aggressively, you are only teaching them to be aggressive as well, how they see you treat and relate to people matters a lot, the kind of relationship they notice between you and your partner is another example they will learn from.

- **Calmness in intervention:** When fights erupt, and you want to intervene, be sure to show a high level of calmness, yelling never solves anything, it only brings about escalation, I know it is really annoying to see your kids getting in a brawl, but be sure to suppress your anger and not show your frustration.

- **Try not to judge and take sides:** When you hear your kids fighting over something (probably a toy), and you get there, with or without an idea of who had it first, try settling the fight regardless, putting blames can build grudges in Kids' minds. It's normal to think about fairness but trust me, the other kid will have the fault too some other time, there you have your balance.

- **Ignorance:** This will be needed at some point, when you find out that your kids start to fight in search of attention, then some amount of ignorance will help make them know that negative attention is not a way of life, because if they are always getting it anytime they fight, then they will keep on doing it anytime attention is needed. Well, a great way to prevent this is to make sure kids have a lot of equal time and attention.

- **Assurance of importance:** This is for older toddler who are having a younger sibling, they believe that with the arrival of the new little one, their significance goes down the drain, they will do almost anything to make sure that doesn't happen, they'll fight for their right. This also requires a lot of attention to the older toddlers so that they can feel secure and not feel threatened by the arrival of the new one. Parents can prevent this by preparing the kid for the new baby, you create a connection even before the baby is born, having them talk to the baby, feel the baby kick, see images of the baby in the belly, can create the desired connection, making them through pictures of their baby days can also help prepare them for what is coming.

- **Verbal lessons:** Try explaining to your kids how bad it is to fight their siblings, show them how they can live together in peace and harmony, you can even encourage them to employ turn taking, it helps reduce the rate of fighting as they know they will have their turns.

Pets

Peaceful co-existence between pets and toddlers depends solely on parents. Toddlers and pets hardly understand each other even though toddlers are always attracted to pets (especially dogs), the parent now must balance and regulate the interactions between them.

It is a different case If the pet has been in the house before the birth of the child, but if you already have a toddler and the plan to get a baby pet comes up, it is advisable to wait until the child grows, because toddlers and baby pets need almost equal amount of attention and care, and having these two together might cause troubles for a parent. Bringing in a grown pet is another different case, that can be easier to handle compared to the case involving a younger aged pet. While other animals too can be brought in as pets, dogs are the most common, followed immediately by cats, mind you, animals that are not in any way compatible with toddlers are reptiles, they are too dangerous to be left around kids.

When introducing the child and the dog, a lot of caution and carefulness is required, there could be a need for a professional dog trainer and the child too has to be taught the dog etiquette, in other words, toddlers are to be taught how to relate with the dog. Parents also have to make sure that toddlers are never left alone with the pets as they might unknowingly do things that can upset the dog's natural instinct, instinct that they don't have control over and are bound to react based on. These incidents would consequentially cause harm to their kids.

Cats, on the other hand, are toddler-friendly too, but can also be dangerous regarding their reactions towards their instinct. They aren't really much different from the dog either in that aspect.

Another thing to be taking seriously is hygiene. Animals, even when regularly taken care of, can harbor germs and diseases, regular cleansing and disinfection of the kids is required as well as for the pets. Take pets to vets regularly for check-up as well as regular all-round check-ups for kids.

Resisting Getting Dressed

Here we go again, another everyday struggle between parents and toddlers, after overcoming the bathroom struggles, the next trouble stage is the dressing. Toddlers can create headaches for parents from very little things, it is up to the parents to get ready and be up to the task. "Tediousness" can be turned to "free off stress" if these following tips are applied duly.

- **Give choices:** This involves giving them the chance to choose between the two clothes you have chosen and presented like, in every other aspect, it gives them the feeling of being in control of the decision making and satisfies their ever-present urge for independence.

- **Patience and calmness:** When kids begin to show resistance and stubbornness, truly, it drives you nuts and tends to trigger your anger senses, but, you are to be careful and suppress that anger that is boiling and pushing to spill out of you, be gentle and patient with them. Your gentle reaction hopefully touches them and calms them down also.

- **Make dress-time fun:** Try being playful while dressing your toddlers, try to make it an enjoyable experience, one which they would always want to happen. You can also get them distracted by offering toys.

- **Be willing to lose:** If the problem is actually the choice of clothes, toddlers can refuse the clothes you have chosen and offered and might want to make their own choices, this especially happens if the kids have favorite clothes, there is no big deal in letting them wear their favorite clothes as long as it is suitable for the weather (even if it means dressing as a superhero or wearing that pajamas to school).

- **A consistently recurring morning routine:** Try repeating the same routine every morning with equally consistent timing. This helps prepare the kids mind for what is to come every morning and can make dress-time a little easier to overcome.

No Kiss for Mom and Dad

Your toddler who usually never gets tired of hugs and kisses, always willing to give or receive, now seem to refuse and reject them, well, that is no reason for alarm, because it is only normal for kids when they're transiting from babies to "big kids." It all comes from the urge to be independent; they now want to feel in control of what happens with them, with your hugs and kisses being part of it. You really have to be patient with them, because this is another stage they have to pass through while growing up, and these hugs and kisses are now of lesser importance to the other things they want to do.

It is advisable to not try and force emotions out of your kids, do not utter condemning words to them as kids are not the manufacturers of their own emotions, you shouldn't make them feel bad for their emotions, because they can't control their emotions like adults. Parents also have to work on their timing, watch the mood of your kids, when they might or might not be open to any, but kids tend to always welcome kisses at bedtime. Also know to stop and not frustrate your kids when you make advances and they refuse, you can try again later, it's harmless to keep trying, just be careful not to annoy them so as not to provoke them into tantrums. Kids who reject hugs and kisses can also have other things that they can be interested in, try tickling, high fives, and others.

Toddlers also show preferences, when they tend to prefer one parent to the other, and in most cases, this tends to favor the mother, since they spend more time with her, so they feel safer with her. Fathers, you don't have to fret at all, it gets better with time, as long as you continue to show your love and affection.

Another case is when boys who are very close to their mothers want to try and detach and give a little space, girls still tend to want to be with their mom a bit more. These are all common cases that are not supposed to cause much perplexity.

Getting Ready for School

Starting school is another important milestone in the life of your kid. When this time comes, different feelings come with it, you are truly excited and joyful at this accomplishment, but this same situation can give you some sort of concern. Onwards, it could be that you are going to spend more time away from each other, another cause for worry could be the fact that you feel your kid is not ready. It is normal for you to think your kid is not ready, this happens with almost every parent, but it is your duty to make sure that your kid is prepared. At two-and-a-half years, pre-schools believe your child is eligible to start, but that doesn't mean that there is an automatic readiness at this age. Before your child can start pre-school, you need to make sure that they have what it takes to thrive in this new world without you.

Tips on How to Get Toddlers Ready for School

- **Separation training:** It's easier for kids who are used to being under the care of a caregiver, you might probably want to do that long before it is time for preschool so that the kid can get used to being away from you from some time. A relative's help can also be employed if you don't want to go with a daycare provider.

- **Self-reliance:** Make sure your kids are already able to handle somethings by themselves, independence is a factor that is needed when kids are starting school. Feeding, toilet training, ability to sleep alone, and all other basics are factors to be considered when kids are starting school.

- **Communication skills:** Listening and speaking skills are required when your kids are starting school, these are factors that will help kids in their learning process. Interaction and socialization with other people will require good communication skills.

- **Encourage learning through play:** Kids' creativity can be enhanced by allowing them to paint and draw. Shape and size recognition can be instilled by letting them play block building and shape sorting. Turn-taking, sharing, and cooperative play can be encouraged by making them take part in organized play with other kids.

- **Reading:** Reading storybooks and other kid books help with your kids' reading abilities.

Additionally, mornings are about to take a new turn, there could be a need to change the usual morning routines. The most significant change might be in the timing, parents might need to change the timing by starting to do things a little earlier in order to prevent lateness.

Kids Cheating Parents

Parents, don't be surprised when you are playing a game (probably a board game for kids) with your toddler, and you notice that she tries to cheat to win the game. Kids are not smart enough to beat us, and they also do not know how bad it is to cheat, so they simply feel that is what they have to do to win the game. Although you might not be able to take it well, but, with your beautiful cheating toddler, you have to be gentle. You are obliged to make them know what they have done is not acceptable, but not with any form of harshness, in fact, you could even make this correction a playful one, but with the assurance that they truly get your message. While playing these games with your kids, you need to try and give them chances of winning, because when they keep loosing, the game becomes boring, leaving them with only two options which is, to leave or to cheat. So, allowing kids to win can prevent cheating in kids, as they grow, the game should get tougher. Also, like I have always said and will keep saying, kids watch us and see the things we do, which they, in turn, replicate, it gives them the feeling that they too can do what every normal human being does. Therefore, you should be sure to set good examples for your kids.

Teaching Parental Values

One of the most important goal a parent aims to achieve in the life of their children is to make sure that they know, have, and display the fundamental moral behavioral values. These values, however, are what defines their personalities in the nearer and farther future, therefore teaching these values to our kids should be top on our priority list. Kids are bound to want to thread the wrong at first, as they are filled with nothing as to what is right or wrong, then it becomes the obligation of the parent to correct them and put them on the right track.

The use of "the three words," please, thank you, and sorry, is the first basic rule that should be taught to kids, using the "please when asking, "thank you" to show appreciation, and "sorry" when it happens that they are wrong. Let them know that nobody is perfect, it is normal for humans to offend each other, but it is important to try to minimize the occurrence. It is also important to let them know that, just saying these words is not enough, they have to really mean it. Politeness is key in everyday interactions with other people.

Other values include integrity, honesty, and keeping true to one's word is essential in our day-to-day lives. Self-discipline; having these commands a lot of respect for a person in the community, kids should be made to know the importance of this. Kids should also learn to be respectful, respect for others, in turn, commands respect for the person. There are still a lot more values, but the above stated can be called the mains, they are like the foundation for all others. This can be easier to achieve when we portray good characters for them to see.

Swearing and Bad Language

With all the excitement and joy that comes with your child reaching the speech milestone, there is also a downside to it. Kids as they learn to speak, also tend to also pick up the negative words, and getting them to stop this habit is not always easy. Kids can copy these words from immediate family members and people around them, from media and the internet, from other kids, even parents can be of influence.

However, you shouldn't be surprised when you hear your kids swearing for the first time, even if you know you are not the swearing type, you are not the only source of knowledge for your kids. Kids use these bad languages for different reasons such as, attention seeking, for fun, to show surprise or shock, to show frustration and anger. Below are some tips on how to handle or curb this habit.

Tips on Handling Swearing and the Use of Bad Languages

- **Refrain from this habit:** Parents that do not want their children to pick up the habit of swearing and bad language usage, should also try to watch their choice of words too, you don't want to be a bad influence to your kids.

- **Don't give them what they want:** Kids can seek attention in many ways, even if it is negative, display of annoyance is also a form of attention to them, so parents should try to exercise patience and calmness when kids do this. In the case of kids using this as a medium to get your attention, parents should try ignoring them, kids would stop using this tactic when they learn that it won't get them any attention. Parents should also make sure to not give kids reasons to desperately seek attention, always create time for your kids, and encourage positive ways of getting your attention.

- **Talk to them:** Let your kids know that swearing is unacceptable, explain to them that some words are not allowed and should not be uttered in daily activities, like when talking to other people, words that can upset them should be avoided. Also, try to provide alternative words that can be used to replace swear words, in the case of expressing surprise. make them know the difference between nice and unpleasant words, and you should always let them know immediately whenever they have used an unpleasant word

- **Deal with the source:** Try to find out the sources where your kids might be getting this influence from, and try to take care of it. Monitor the media exposure of your child, make use of parental control features in gizmos, so that they will be restricted to only programs meant for their ages. If you find out that your kids are learning from other kids, try calling the attention of the kids' parents to the situation, so that all the kids would be corrected. Ask other members of the family to try and caution their speech around the kids.

- **Praise for progress:** Try showing appreciation by praising your kids when you notice changes in their expressions, it gets them to use the right words more often.

In addition, be careful not to encourage this habit by smiling or laughing when your kids use these words, even if it's funny to you. Make yourself a better person too by limiting the usage of these foul languages.

You are the Best

The words we say to our kids go a really long way in their lives psychologically, parents should try taking their time to give their kids words of praise and encouragement, every little chance we get, never hesitate to dish out these words. Praises bring out good manners in kids, and encouraging words have a positive effect on the self-esteem of kids, self-confidence takes a boost in the presence of motivations. Words like, *"You are the best"*, *"you are strong"*, *"you are powerful"*, *"you are wise"*, *"you are valuable"*, *"you are kind"*, *"you are a blessing"*, *"you are creative"*, *"I believe in you"*, *"I have faith in you"*, *"it's okay to make mistakes, everybody does every now and then"*, *"you are a great helper"*, *"you are excellent at..."*, *"I appreciate it when you..."*

Just uttering these words isn't enough, make sure you truly mean it when you say them, kids are not stupid, they can tell when you don't mean what you say too. Apart from the psychological aspects, showing this attitude towards your kids also make them know how you feel about them.

Lastly, although not the least, kids' output is based on the input, what they get is what they give out, this attitude becomes part of them too. Kids that get appreciated a lot become very appreciative people because they already know the value of appreciation.

Hobbies and Creativity

Hobbies and creativity, these two works hand in hand, and are present in the lives of all kids. Every kid always has some sort of obsession, there is always a particular thing that they are intensely interested in more than others. Sometimes, it could be activities such as painting and drawing, building and arranging blocks, puzzle solving and so on, and sometimes kids could be interested in fantasies such as fairies, mermaids and underwater creatures, superheroes, some of their cartoon characters, etc. It is also possible for kids to be involved in the two categories, happens a lot. Toddler-age hobbies are not necessary determinants of what they will want to be in future, as on a lot of occasions, these interests tend to fade away as they grow older, but at the same time, some adults today that are excelling in their fields started from their tender ages. The most deciding factor is the actions the parents take in handling their interests, whether the kids grow or deteriorate in these abilities, most times depends on the parents.

Some hobbies can also be parent-infused, kids can follow in the footsteps of their parents and become interested in what parents expose them to. For example, A kid that helps parents in the garden might want to pick up an interest in the field, kids whose parent are football-enthusiastic can end up loving football. Other hobbies can just come from natural tender-age child's play, like painting and drawing, kids generally, when in possession of a paper and pen just destroy--decorate the jotter, kids can stain anywhere with anything that produces color, if this type of kids are allowed to continue in this act (but with the supervision and monitoring of parents), they can pick up an interest in this line. Parents, however, need to discover, understand, and foster these creative interests. Below are some tips on how to encourage toddlers' hobbies and creativity.

- **Create a comfortable and conducive atmosphere:** Help your kids by creating an environment that supports their interests. Your support and encouragement motivate them and make them feel comfortable with what they are doing, knowing fully well that they are fully supported. When they make mistakes, make sure to be there for them, encourage them, and make them know it is normal for mistakes to occur, offer motivation, so they don't lose interest.

- **Avoid rewards:** Do not reward your kids for being creative, it adds pressure and makes them to always want to impress, this will contaminate the main motive of just exploring and expressing themselves.

- **Exposure:** Expose them to accomplished examples pertaining to their line of interest. For kids who like football, take them to watch football matches, let them join coaching schools, or for kids who prefer artistic works, cover your walls and decorate your tables with different artworks, and so on. This gives them more insight into these topics, as well as consolidating their interests.

- **Discussions:** Bring up conversations with your kids about their line of interest. There are many ways by which you can discuss these things, you can ask about how they feeling while in the act, you can ask them to come up with new ideas, but be careful not to judge their ideas, don't tell them if one idea is good or not, except of course if it is dangerous, then explain gently to them.

- **Freedom to be creative:** Be sure to allow your kids some space, give them the space to be creative and don't try to choose for them, or order them to do what you feel they should. Let them be in control of the situation.

- **Provide space and resources:** Kids should be provided with the necessary equipment, soccer balls with football boots and jerseys, paintbrush, and colors with drawing pencils and pads, and so on, can be provided, and set aside a specific space for them to carry out their activities to give them freedom and protect the other places from disorder.

Part Three
Particularity of Every Age

The development of kids varies with ages, in this chapter, I'll talk about the different phases of growth and development with particularity to each age from one to five. You should expect largely to see what mostly happens in every one of these years. You are more or less going to see what you should be expecting when your kids reach these ages and how they can be handled. Although the group "toddler" really refers to children of ages one to three, we will also extend a little bit into the life of preschoolers, which are of ages four and five. So, in essence, we will be talking about the life of kids from their first year to the fifth. This chapter will be divided into two sections: Section one is made up of years one to three where they are toddlers, while section two will be the extension into the life of their immediate seniors of ages four and five.

Section One
Toddlers

An insight into the first, second, and third years of toddlers.

One Year Old

The end of the beginning is here, with what I call the "beginning" being the first twelve months. Now when you look back to the time you gave birth to that innocent, helpless, little baby, and compare it to the present day, you find that a lot of changes have taken place in your little one, well, meanwhile, the major changes have barely started. As much as it is the end of the beginning, this is also another beginning. It is the first of all the milestones your child is going to reach, it is the first major birthday your kid will be having. This is the point where your child leaves baby or infanthood to become a toddler, and at this point is where your toddler begins to grow and develop in many aspects, your toddler begins to toddler-versions of human characteristics. I'll be giving insights on what you should be expecting in the subsequent twelve months in the following section.

Motor skills. Now as the name toddler implies (toddler literally means a child that toddles, with toddle meaning to walk unsteadily), although, walking at this stage is not guaranteed, as this is when the whole "toddling" thing begins, kids can at least stand on their feet without help, and before now, they would have gone through the crawling stage, and by their eighteenth month, the unsteady walking should have begun. With the arms not to go unmentioned, there is also an upgrade in the arm-strength which increases their ability to apply force when needed. Sitting without help is another feature of the improved gross motors skills.

Having discussed the gross motor skills, fine motor skills are next up. This aspect refers to the coordination of the eyes with the hands and fingers. This is said to happen earlier than the gross motor skills, so before the twelfth month, your kid should have begun holding small objects, turning book pages, and the likes, other advanced ones get to come in gradually.

However, if these things can happen a little earlier or later, this should not be a cause for alarm, the time differs from kid to kid, but if you observe that it is out of range, then you might want to let your pediatrician know. To say the truth, this information will be better passed by the pediatrician, so you need to make enquires way before this time (if the doctor hasn't discussed it yet).

Communication and language skills. This includes improvement in speaking skills and the use of sign language. Kids who, with all the effort they put in trying to speak, were only blabbers will now show some obvious improvements in their speeches, where words like dada, mama, no, and some other elementary words, have formed out of the previous gibberish. Here, kids also learn to use and understand simple sign languages, the one that most commonly comes first being head-nodding, then there could be other signs like touching of genitals to show that they are pressed, making thirst gestures, and so on. Apart from expressing themselves, they also understand these gestures and word, they already have a full understanding of the nodding gestures and can differentiate a "yes" nod from a "no" nod.

Cognitive skills. Although it might not be sharp yet, a little mental processing-ability should be noticed. They now understand that some things, even if not seen, are still in existence. Therefore, they can now know to search for things that are not directly seen, probably under one or two covers or behind an obstacle.

Physical growth. Kids, at one-year-old, go through an obvious growth and development in their body, they obviously grow very big compared to when they were given birth to. There is also a significant growth in the size of the brain (this is especially responsible for the development of their cognitive skills). So be prepared for a wardrobe change, they are definitely going to outgrow the old ones.

Also, parents should try and tend to their explorational needs, because, at this stage, kids begin to explore their environment and the world they're just coming to understand. Try creating an exploration-aiding environment. Also, as always, healthcare is very important, be sure to take them to pediatricians regularly for thorough check-ups, and vaccination should be taken seriously. All the baby-proof security measures should still be intact for safety reasons, they are still babies, you know.

Two Years Old

So, now that the first year is gone, your toddler is on course of becoming a big kid, and there are significant developments in every aspect of their lives. There is an improvement on the developments that have occurred at age one,

Communication: Speaking becomes clearer, two-year-olds are now able to say a three-word long sentence, an upgrade to their one year younger self, don't be surprised when you see your two-year-old singing the songs you sing to them.

Movement: Walking becomes steadier, with a significant balance in the heels and toes usage. Kids at two already begin to run, of course, when you pass the walking stage, why not go for running, right? Straight to the next level. They also do a lot of climbing, from furniture to playground equipment, as long as it looks climbable (to them), they can climb up and down. Pulling toys along while walking is also common among kids around this age, since they are now bigger in size, and are steady on their feet, they now have the power to pull things along while they move (depends on weight).

Hands and Fingers: Spontaneous scribbling, another feature in kids at this age, the ability to build towers of three or more blocks is also present. An upgrade to that of "year one."

Cognition: Cognition is improved to the point that imagination now comes into play, and they can now engage in make-believe (imaginative) plays, they begin to recognize and discern differences in shapes and colors.

Of course, there is continuous growth and development in different parts of the body, and as they grow, they grow to become independent, they now begin to feel that natural urge for independence. At this stage they begin to develop a sense of control that, if not given, can be a cause for power struggles, tantrums, and the likes, they tend to want to feed themselves, dressing themselves (although with clothes that are easy for them to handle), they can even get to be choosy about what to eat, and this comes from the fact that they want to imitate older kids or adults, and soothe themselves with the feeling of doing things by themselves. This age also comes with the sense of fear, while younger kids might not have this issue, fear can begin to set in at around the age of two, kids can have different and random reasons for fear, monster under the bed, fear of spiders, fear of the dark are just a few of many fear factors for kids, Its left in the hands of the parents to help them handle these fears (refer to part two, "monsters under the bed"). This also is a really good time to introduce toilet training (of course, without pushing). Good luck with the "terrible twos."

Three Years Old

Welcome to the "threenagers." Growth still continues, although not as rapid as in the previous years, there is still a continuous improvement in the foundation laid in the first year, traits are very stronger. Children at this stage can begin cooperative play (play involving other kids) as opposing to solo play where every kid plays alone, even if they are beside each other. This is the bridge between toddler-age and the preschool-age, this is more or less the age where toddlers officially become preschoolers because they already begin to have a better understanding of how different things work. Movement ability gets to its peak around this age, steady walking is no more a news, they can now even go up and down the stairs without help, walk, run, jump, the complete package is present. Three-year-olds will ask you more questions, they need your help to satisfy their curiosity as they begin to explore the world around them. Exploration expands as they grow, and at this age, the rate is very high, parents should help enhance their creativity by providing an exploration and expression aiding environment (refer to part two, "hobbies and creativity").

Parents should make it an obligation to make sure that kids have been taught to express their discomfort or displeasure with words rather than throwing tantrums. Kids of this age are also said to understand emotions, they show emotions and sympathy, don't be surprised when you see your three-year-old giving hugs when they see other kids or friends (yes, they now have friends). Also, kids, around this time, should have shown their preferred hand.

If your kid hasn't yet been potty-trained, now is more of the perfect time to get it into them, there should be no case of unreadiness, kids at this age are mostly ready to be toilet-trained. This age group should also be able to handle not very demanding dressing, for example, you don't expect them to lace their own shoes, or put on their own belts (dress or trousers), but they can at least put on their socks.

There can also be a lot of limit-testing, they sometimes want to know what happens as a result of their action, they also tend to test limits if it sparks any kind of reaction from, so when this happens, parents should play smart and don't give them what they want, try the ignorance method so that they don't get the impression that they can always get your attention with limit testing. Don't forget, your kid is transiting from a baby to a big kid, a little bit of strictness is required to make them know what is wrong from what is right, as this is basically what builds their adult-personality.

Section Two

Preschoolers

Now that we know what to expect of our toddlers, its time to talk about our big kids. In the previous section, it has been made known that the third year is said to be the middle or transition age, they are more or less sitting on the fence and are neither fully toddlers nor fully preschoolers as this is where toddler-age ends and preschool-age begins. We will proceed to talk about our preschool-school-age kids.

Four Years Old

L ike the third year being the bridge between toddlerhood and preschool-age, this is also the season where your kid becomes a big kid, what a big difference in a short time, just a little over 500 days ago, your big kid was still a toddler. Parent. Kudos! You have scaled through all the time they were babies, "terrible twos," and "threenagers," but don't celebrate just yet trust me, it never really gets easier, along with a whole lot of "ups," comes a whole lot of "downs." Meet the "frustrating fours":

Now, you can refer to your kid as a pre-kindergartener, as that the main milestone that is commonly reached at this age, your kids is now more than ready to start preschool. Starting school can be really hard for kid (and even parents), if they are not used to being away from their parents, so parents should be sure to prepare kids properly beforehand by making them spend time with other caregivers, could be daycare groups, could be relatives (be careful with whom you leave your kid with though), that will prepare them for when the time comes, they get to know that they will have to be somewhere that you won't be for some part of the day, and later, you are coming to pick them up. Also, help your kids to love learning so that they will be prepared for the life ahead, this is easier to pull off when play is involved, as learning through play is very crucial.

Expect some maturity, there is more cooperation among peers where they now share their toys with other kids and turn-taking is practiced, they allow for negotiations to resolve conflicts, there are more creativity and imagination in fantasy plays, a good show of self-control, etc. Four-year-olds ask questions a lot, you should be expecting a whole lot of "why" questions, and it is very important to help your kid learn. I know it can be very frustrating at times, but again, and as always, you'll need a lot of patience. Parents are also required to help their kids deal with their fears (all the "monsters under the bed," "fear of the dark," etc.), if their highly imaginative brain can create fantasies, then it can also produce frightening imaginations, thereby bringing about the fears we are talking about.

Strong-Willed Four-Year-Olds

Four-year-olds are good at testing limits, but parents should be well prepared after reading the parts one and two of this book. Although there are naturally strong-willed kids, this usually happens more when they are around this age. Strong-willed kids need to be dealt with patiently but strictly so as to not give them the impression that they can always have their way. A quick reminder on handling a "four-year-old" kid:

- *Be calm patient, yelling never solves but impounds*

- *Verbal Reprimand is necessary*

- *Ignore attention-seeking misbehaviors*

- *Use timeouts*

- *Appreciate good behavior by praising*

- *Follow through with consequences on broken rules*

- *It's okay to remove privileges*

- *Never give in*

- *Offer allowable choices, to give control*

- *Lead by example, don't do one thing and ask another*

Bullying

One problem kids can face is bullying, and this is very delicate and difficult to handle. If you notice that your kid is involved in any form of bullying, it's best to talk to your kid about it, ask your kid to narrate how it happened (or has been happening) and praise your kid for talking to you about it, this will make them feel safer, do not give them impressions that will make them feel like they are weak or inferior, for example, you don't say words like "you poor little thing", "you should learn how to stand up and fight for yourself", etc. You then, contact your kid's teacher and report the issue, don't take matter into your hands by going directly to the bully-kid or the parent, this won't solve the problem and can consequently cause more problems, the schools will know how to deal with the case. If talking to the teacher does not change anything, then, you might need to file a formal complaint to the school authority, meetings can be set up, there is no need to be aggressive, be calm and cooperative in order to come up with a good solution to the problem. If the school then ultimately does nothing to change the situation, then I will advise you to withdraw your kid and get another school with a better anti-bully setup.

As much as different kids grow at different rates, it is still required to see a pediatrician when you notice some setback or very slow growth in your kids.

Five Years Old

The official "big kid" age. Growth and development continue as usual, and there are more milestones reached, they grow more independent, but no matter how much they can do on their own, there is still a need for attention and assistance. Parents need to be present in their kids world, this can be achieved by spending special quality time together every day, you could set a particular time for this, and you can engage in activities like playing together, watching tv together (be careful to not exceed the recommended screen-time limit), reading a book, or just spend one-on-one time, this creates connection, which gets stronger by the day, between you two.

Rules should be kept simple, as they are known for following rules now that they have a better understanding of how things work, but when the rules are too complex or excessive, then it tends to piss them off. Give full support and encouragement to enhance their creativities or activities, parents can even allow kids start professional trainings on their preferred activities (sports, dancing, drumming, etc.) at this age (remember people like Serena & Venus Williams, Lionel Messi, and others).

Educationally, at this stage, your five-year-old kids should already be conversant with simple additions and subtractions, as this age, he/ she has been taught in the pre-kindergarten classes as they are supposed to have at age four. This is the general minimum age that has been stated for kids to start kindergarten/preschool classes. Encourage your kids to play with other kids, plays involving turn taking, energy-involving activities like running, swinging, playing soccer, board games, all have a part to play in your kid's life.

As understanding as your five years old might be, kids will still be kids, so there could be some defiance and disobedience, they won't always do what you want them to do. This is surely frustrating and exhausting because this is not just tantrums anymore, this is an advanced limit-testing, in which the kids now knows more of what they are doing. Whining is another unpleasant feature at this age, kids this age can be really pestering, they don't always want to hear a "no", when you say that, they just resort to whining believing persistent begging can be used to get parents persuaded into changing their minds, this also can be really frustrating. Don't let it hit as a surprise when you detect lying in your kid, kids can also make up imaginative stories to get you to do what they want, they can also lie to get out of trouble. After all, Lying isn't that hard. Here are some few tips on dealing with a five-year-olds unwanted behavior.

- **Verbal information:** Let them know what and what is not accepted

- **Set Limits:** Set certain limits that restrict them from doing the unaccepted, and be sure to support with reasonable consequences that are directly enforced when lines are crossed.

- **Be understanding:** Be gentle with your reprimands, do a little consolation afterward, try to understand how they will feel and show it. For example, after forcing to bed, let her know you know how it feels to be asked to do what one doesn't want to, but let her know that it just really had to be done.

- **Release control:** It is always advisable to let kids feel in control, makes it a lot easier to get them to do things.

- **Provide alternatives:** Instead of just asking them to stop kicking the ball (around the room), you can provide an alternative place to kick the ball, like going outside.

- **Employ timeouts:** Timeouts give kids time to cool and reflect on incidents, it prevents scene creation, and help them act better next time.

- **Promote good behavior:** Try not to make them feel any worse after a bad behavior, this might only get them to only force good behavior, it's not really of their own will. Instead, only highlight and praise good behaviors, that urges them to behave better to get more praises.

12 Basic Rules of Education of a Baby

Parenting can be hilarious, it's like bringing a pandora's box and a Santa's bag, and emptying the content into one big container. Parenting, with all the joy and good feeling it brings, is still very frustrating, and if clueless, can be really impossible. The life of a child is largely dependent on the parents, so parents need to be really careful not to take any actions (or inactions) that will negatively affect the lives of kids. For the achievement of successful parenthood, here the basic rule a parent must follow.

- **Love and affection can't be too much:** There can never be too much love from you to your kids, it's like the main reason why you are their parent, no one else has the right to love them better, unending love is what is expected of you to your kids. Make sure to express your love at every opportunity you get, from physical expressions (hugs and kisses) to emotional (in your words), you should never hold back, it's not too much if your child receives nothing less than ten hugs in a day (could be more). Some parents might fear that showing so much love can have a spoiling effect on their kids, which is wrong, what actually does that are the actions parents take in the name and place of "love," like material indulgences, lowered expectations, leniency, etc. Children can spot the difference between when you are showing genuine love, and when you're just trying to "bribe" them. The latter is what actually spoils them, but in the case of the former, they can feel safe and protected.

- **Time and attention:** You should never be too busy to give your kids ample time and attention, create time to play together, have fun times, and make sure to attend to every one of their needs. Quality time with kids creates a good parent-kid connection and enhances a cordial relationship. This, in turn, makes kids want to please their parents.

- **Good Communication and understanding:** There should be regular communication between parents and kids. Parents should try and create a communicative atmosphere around the home, where kids and parents can freely express themselves with ultimate respect for every member of the house-even toddlers should be regarded as individuals and treated with respect. It is also important for parents to understand their kids and vice versa, this also enhances good relationship between parents and kids.

- **Rules and limits:** Make rules and set limits. Make sure that rules are reasonable and followable, followed up by consequences that are potent but are not extreme attached. Also, know how to connect consequences to offenses. Rules should be well explained to kids to be sure of a full understanding so that kids won't have to pay for what they know nothing about.

- **Flexibility:** Every kid is different from another in character and every other thing, though, some parenting styles are more preferable to other, there is still a need for parents to be flexible in their parenting styles and delve a little bit into every type when necessary. Parents have to study and understand their kids and try to adjust their parenting style to suit their personalities.

- **Learn from experience:** The best teacher in life is experience, be it from yours or from others, if this isn't your first kid, then you probably have had some experience by now, this is definitely useful, although kids are not all the same, there will still be some times where the experience you have will come in handy. If you're having a baby for the first time, then you'll need some help from those that have been there before you. Never be shy or afraid to ask questions from experts and professionals, whatever baffles you, make sure you ask.

- **Only reinforce good behavior:** Do not make references to kids' bad behaviors, when there is much attention paid to this, they tend to do it more often. Instead, only do that for good behaviors, so that that' is what settles into their subconscious, then, that's what they get to do often.

- **Reflection:** This means looking back at your own childhood, it involves reviewing your own childhood and how your parents did their parenting, you pick the positivity part, look at the inadequate ones and see how you can improve on those aspects. Reflecting on your childhood can help in training your kid greatly, more than you will think.

- **Enhance your kids' independence:** This occurs naturally, kids at some point, demand some autonomy and have the urge to do things independently. Parents are tempted to always think, kids are too small to handle some things, but the truth is that parents should allow them to do somethings for themselves, even if it is imperfect (which it will). This enhances self-dependence, boosts self-confidence, and esteem, it also gives them the mind to want to try new things.

- **Patience is key:** The ability to be calm in a hot atmosphere, being able to hold back aggressive and negative anger expressions like yelling, spanking and the likes, is a quality every parent should have. These actions only escalate issues and hardening the already difficult task of managing kids' temper and emotional outpours.

- **Lead by example:** What you do is very important, how you treat others, how you react in situations, your habits, things you say, things you do in general affects the characters, behaviors, and personalities of kids. They more or less copy and paste our traits, so be careful to not give your kids the wrong impression, orientation, and perspective of life.

- **Consistency:** Another key quality parents need to have is being consistent, this includes appreciations and reprimands, when you do one thing today and do the other tomorrow in the same circumstance, they will get confused and not know what is accepted or not, for example, if you take away the food as a consequence to food flinging today, and tomorrow the kid throws food again but you do nothing, you are confusing the kid, but when you repeat the deed again the next time, the kid then knows, that is the consequence for throwing and wasting food, there is a chance that the act will stop or significantly reduce a whole lot.

These above-stated points, with how simple they might look, are very important and can be really challenging, parenting and parenthood is not a bed of roses, but they can go a really long way in training your kids.

Money Lesson for Toddlers

From age four, parents can begin given kids lessons about money. At this stage, they are not too young to know about money. Kids with the wrong orientation about money tend to have poor financial managerial skills. Some constituents of money lessons include,

Saving habits

Contentment

Giving spirit

Avoiding impulse purchase

Money is to be worked for

The usefulness of opportunity cost; ability to prioritize needs

Budget making and planning

Teach entrepreneurship

Leading by example is also very vital so that our kids can learn from us. You can encourage saving by getting piggy banks for them and helping them inculcate the habit. You can also get three jars with each jar serving different purposes of saving, giving, and spending, this is a 3-in-1 method to encourage the three mentioned lessons.

Bonus

Here's your bonus

<< http://marysimmonsbook.com/home/ >>

About The Author

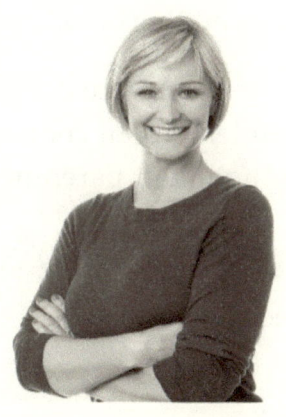

Mary Simmons graduated from Boston University in the faculty of social psychology and devoted herself to studying the problems of the relationship between children and adults, and has participated in research. As a member of several associations in Boston she aims at improving relations between children and has written articles on the upbringing of children in magazines and online publications. Mary has three children: 12, 5 and 2 years old. She sees her strongest achievement in sharing her own experience and skills to other people.

Please, Leave a Review!

I hope you enjoyed this book!

Reviews from awesome customers like you help others to feel confident about choosing this book too and navigate through their parenting times safely.

Please take a minute to share your experience!

I really appreciate it !